I0509981

HOW TO FIND CARE FOR YOUR ELDERLY PARENT

**A guide to selecting assisted living,
nursing home and
what to do when
the money runs out**

By

Kady Dash

Notice of rights

Copyright © 2020 by Kady Dash. All rights reserved.

No part of this publication may be reproduced, stored in a retrieval system, or transmitted in any form or by any means, electronic, mechanical, photocopying, recording, scanning, or otherwise, without the prior written permission of the author.

Limit of Liability/Disclaimer of Warranty: While the publisher and author have used their best efforts in preparing this book, they make no representations or warranties with respect to the accuracy or completeness of the contents of this book and specifically disclaim any implied warranties of merchantability or fitness for a particular purpose. No warranty may be created or extended by sales representatives or written sales materials. The advice and strategies contained herein may not be suitable for your situation. You should consult with a professional when appropriate. Neither the publisher nor the author shall be liable for any loss of profit or any other commercial damages, including but not limited to special, incidental, consequential, personal, or other damages.

CONTENTS

How to find care for your elderly parent	1
Introduction	9
Time to take action	10
Difficult conversations	12
A durable power of attorney	14
In-person visits are a must	16
A Place for Mom	19
The place for my mom	21
Medicaid nuts and bolts	23
Medical assessment	25
Signing the papers	27
Did I make a big mistake?	29
Life in an assisted living facility	32
Three months warning	35
Orchestrating the transfer from the assisted living facility to the nursing home	38
Rooms in the nursing home	41

Admission to the nursing home	43
Other provisions to be on the lookout for	46
Resident payments	48
Initial Medicaid application	51
Application questions clarifications	54
Timeline for processing the Medicaid application	63
Request for additional information	65
Difficulties getting information as the power of attorney	69
When a power of attorney has no power	72
Missing the deadline	76
The denial	78
Medical assessment	82
The approval	83
Annual re-certifications	85
Lifeline program	86
Senior care options plans	88
Interview questions	90
Questions to ask assisted living facilities	92
Questions to ask when selecting Nursing Homes	113
Conclusion	123
Appendix	125
Summary of documents you will need	131

| Alphabetical Index | 134 |
| Books By This Author | 135 |

INTRODUCTION

This book is the helping hand I wish I had had when I was navigating through the maze of options for taking care of an aging parent with dementia. In this book, I concentrate on practical issues starting with selecting the right facility, knowing what questions to ask during the visits, and on the step-by-step process of what you need to do when the money to pay for the accommodations your parent needs runs out. By the end of my search, I had compiled a comprehensive list of questions that you should cover when selecting a facility. These questions are part of this book. I include not only the questions, but also the answers based on my specific experience so you will have a basis for comparison. Not thinking of all these questions in advance made me worry more and made the decisions harder to make. I hope you can benefit from my experience and be confident in your choices.

TIME TO TAKE ACTION

I had seen the signs of my mother's declining memory and ability to think logically for a few years. I took over paying her bills and got helpers who would do her grocery shopping. The realization that things were coming to a crisis happened when I received a phone call from the police in the town where my mother lived. The officer told me my mother had been calling the station several times a week to report thefts in her home. She was reporting the theft of knives, forks, toothbrushes, scissors, and other small household items that would not interest any thief.

The problem was that she was misplacing things, and, when she could not find them, the only logical explanation to her was that someone was stealing them. I found most of the lost items (and they often

HOW TO FIND CARE FOR YOUR ELDERLY PARENT

were in odd places), but could not convince her that the items were not being stolen. To avoid potential thefts, she started hiding her favorite things. Unfortunately, this only exacerbated the problem as she could not recall where she hid these items or even that she did, in fact, hide them. The final straw that made me realize that life could not continue as before was when she thought I was someone else. She began talking about me, with me, but was referring to me in the third person.

Tip:

>*When talking to other children of people with dementia, I found that they also encountered situations where their parents explained misplaced household items by theft. So, be on the lookout for these symptoms, especially if the "stolen" items are everyday household items of little value. If these situations occur over and over again, it is time to take action.*

DIFFICULT CONVERSATIONS

I often heard that people with dementia do not know they have it. My mother could not put a name to her problem, but she knew that something was wrong. When I told her that I was worried about her living on her own, she agreed. Mom said she wanted me to find her a place where she could get help with daily chores like meal preparation and cleaning. I thought she also needed reminders so that she would take her medications on time.

I immediately started looking for assisted living places. I have prepared a list of questions I asked every place I visited so I could compare different facilities. As I learned more about the assisted living and nursing homes, I continued to add new questions to the list. By the time I started writing this book, the list of questions has grown to eighty. Even

HOW TO FIND CARE FOR YOUR ELDERLY PARENT

if you don't ask all eighty questions during your search, I hope the topics will give you eighty things to think about as you make your decisions.

A DURABLE POWER OF ATTORNEY

A durable power of attorney is an essential document for every caregiver. This document allows you to make decisions on behalf of your parents. If you have a power of attorney, you can pay bills on behalf of your parents and direct their medical care. Note that the word "durable" is critical because the non-durable power of attorney automatically ends when the person becomes incapacitated.

Even though the ability to make medical decisions is usually included in the general power of attorney, it is best to also have an explicit medical power of attorney paperwork, the health care proxy. This document designates a person as the primary decision maker if a person is facing life and death circumstances. In this document, your parent chooses a person who will make choices about treatment options, insurance benefits, and life support.

It is best to create these documents when your parent is well and does not need help making decisions. Life is unpredictable, and it is smart to have legal paperwork in place before it is required.

My mother saw a lawyer and created both documents 20 years ago. She gave me the original documents for safekeeping. When I needed to use the paperwork, many institutions required me to show them the original and only then accepted a copy for their records. She did everything right, and only now, I realized how fortunate I am that she thought of it. The fact that the documents were 20 years old was not an issue.

IN-PERSON VISITS ARE A MUST

I visited half a dozen assisted living facilities within a 15-minute drive from my house. I did not like any of them. Some of them looked very decrepit. In other facilities, residents looked like zombies. In yet other places, the sales pitch was so intense that the environment did not feel right. I found one facility that I really liked, but it had a waiting list, so I had to strike it off my list.

One of the key questions on my list was what would happen when my mother ran out of funds. She had enough savings to cover about two years in an assisted living facility. Some places did not accept residents who could not prove they could pay for many years of residency. Some facilities provided a few beds for people with limited funds. These beds are paid for by private or state money (i.e., non-medicaid funds). The number of such rooms is limited, and they have a waiting list. The facilities with subsidized rooms could not guarantee a spot for a specific period of time. For example, they could not promise that my mother would have a room available to her in two years.

Some facilities took part in "adult foster care," a program aimed at low-income residents. I was not familiar with adult foster care programs. I learned that they are similar to assisted living where care is provided for an individual in a facility with shared living and dining areas. However, there are some important differences. They offer only non-medical assistance (that is., they do not have skilled nursing staff) and there is not 24-hour access to awake staff. In foster care, there is 24-hour access to staff, but they are asleep at night. In assisted living, there is 24-hour access to awake and on-duty staff.

The cost of adult foster care is approximately half of the cost of nursing home care, and in most cases, it is also a less expensive option than assisted living. Neither Medicare nor Medicare Supplemental insurance cover assisted living or foster care. However, if you receive Medicaid and need help with at least one activity of daily living, Group Adult Foster Care (GAFC) may cover the cost of personal care services if you live in a GAFC-certified facility. However, GAFC pays only for personal care expenses, and does not cover room and board. Note that not all facilities accept GAFC, so you need to ask explicitly if this option is available.

Because my mother had some savings, it made the situation more complicated. I had to make plans for two scenarios, what to do while she could pay for her room and board and what would happen when the money ran out.

The places I visited during my first round of visits did not offer a clear explanation of what would happen after she ran out of money. The facility representatives told me that they could not guarantee that she could stay in the same facility when her funds were exhausted. This statement meant that I would have to start the search for a new facility again when she spent all her savings. It also meant I would need to put my mother through another move two years down the road. A change of surroundings is traumatic for a person with dementia, as they often find it difficult to remember the new surroundings and new people.

A PLACE FOR MOM

I heard ads for a service called "A Place for Mom," and at the start of my search, I looked at their website and did not like it. The site did not provide any specific information online, you had to register and call them on the phone. I was afraid of getting endless solicitation calls from the service, and so I started the search on my own without using their service. After not finding a facility that I liked, out of desperation, I phoned "A Place for Mom." I described the situation to them, including the fact that she would run out of money in two years. They recommended two places for me. I visited both and really liked one of them. After the initial contact with the service, I only had one more phone call from "A Place for Mom." They wanted to know if either of the places they recommended was a match. I told them I would follow up with one home they recommended. I said I would contact them if I needed more help. They never tried to sell me anything else.

About a year later, I mentioned to the director of the assisted living home that I found their facility through "A Place for Mom." I confessed to him I was pleasantly surprised that they were helpful, free, and did not continue to bother me with marketing phone calls. He said that even though the service was free to me, the assisted living facility pays "A Place for Mom" to refer people to them. I thought it would be useful to note that "A Place for Mom" is not an unbiased independent service. They are working for the assisted living facilities that contract with them, and those are the facilities they recommend to people who contact them. I found "A Place for Mom" very helpful, and I used their recommendation, but they did not disclose their financial connection to the places they recommended.

THE PLACE FOR MY MOM

The facility I liked was a small family-owned facility with 40 residents in assisted living and about 100 residents in the nursing home. The assisted living facility and the nursing home were in adjacent buildings connected via locked doors. During my visit, they showed me both facilities. The residents in both assisted living and the nursing home looked alert, and I even talked to a couple of them. Most of the rooms in the assisted living facility were single-person studio apartments. Most of the rooms in the nursing home were double occupancy.

The price for a double occupancy rooms in the assisted living (that is., a room with a roommate) was approximately $1,000 cheaper per month. The savings on a double occupancy room did not seem to be large enough to warrant this option. I felt that a single occupancy room would be a smoother transition from independent living to an assisted living home.

One of my concerns, based on visits to other facilities, was that the staff would force my mother to participate in games and other social activities. She has never been a social person, and I knew that if they tried to force her to become one, it would be difficult for her. Unlike the other places, the staff told me they would not try to force my mother into social activities if she did not want to take part in them.

Unlike other assisted living facilities, this place gave me a reasonable answer about what would happen when my mother's money ran out.

The explanation I received from the assisted living director (next chapter details his explanation) let me feel that there was a path forward. I liked the facility, I liked the people I spoke with, and I thought I had a general outline of what will happen when the money runs out.

The only negative for this facility was that it was further away from my house than I wanted, but I liked everything else about it. So I had to compromise on the driving distance.

MEDICAID NUTS AND BOLTS

The assisted living director explained that Medicaid does not cover assisted living, but Medicaid does cover nursing homes.

To qualify for Medicaid, a person must qualify both medically and financially. To qualify medically, the person either needs nursing facility skilled level of care, or have a medical or mental condition that requires a small amount of skilled nursing help but substantial assistance with daily living activities. A skilled level of care means needing injections, wound care, catheter care, or other medical needs. Assistance with daily activities includes help with bathing, dressing, toileting, eating, or mobility.. This assistance must be needed at least three times a week.

Note that a dementia diagnosis on its own does not qualify a person for a nursing home. However, many dementia patients do qualify, as they need help with daily activities. Once the Medicaid office receives an application, they send a nurse to evaluate the individual's level of ability to carry out everyday tasks.

To qualify financially for Medicaid coverage, an individual must have no more than $2,000 in resources ($3,000 for a married couple). Resources include all assets including savings and property with two exceptions. In Massachusetts, one car of any value is exempt, as long as a household member is using it. The home is exempt up to an equity value of $878,000 (in 2019) if one of the spouses lives in the house or if the resident plans to return to it. Note that the rules in different states might be different. All the specifics in this book are based on my personal experience in the Commonwealth of Massachusetts.

I included a link to information for other states in Appendix at the end of this book.

MEDICAL ASSESSMENT

The next step was for the nurse to visit my mother and evaluate her condition. The director explained that they needed to know if she could live in an assisted living facility or required a nursing home. The nurse determined that my mother currently could function with the level of help that assisted living provides. At the end of the evaluation, she warned me that dementia is a progressive condition, and with time, my mother would need more and more assistance. I asked the nurse to give me her projection of my mother's condition in two years. She could only speak in generalities based on the initial assessment and her experience with other patients. She said that my mother's current tests were marginal. Given the progressive nature of dementia, my mother would likely do worse on the tests in two years. This means that as time passed, she would likely fail the tests and probably medically qualify for the nursing home. She told me they would evaluate her health every six months and communicate with me about her status. Everything felt right, and I expressed interest in having my mother move into their facility.

Looking back, the nurse's assessment of the progressive nature of my mother's disease was pretty accurate. For example, my mother's ability to take the medications with only light prompting has evaporated. Early on, she would take medication at prescribed times after the attendants reminded her. Towards the end of her stay in the assisted living, my mother began refusing to take her medication. Even though this negatively affected her health, the assisted living staff was not allowed to take action to help. The staff in the assisted living facility can only remind residents about medicine; they are not qualified to try to convince them to take it. Once she moved to the nursing home, the nurses were able to do some extra coaxing, and she began taking her medications again on a more regular basis.

SIGNING THE PAPERS

After the nurse finished my mother's assessment, the assisted living facility asked me to come back to select the room and sign the paperwork. They let me pick an apartment out of three options. I chose a studio on the second floor with a beautiful view of trees and a Koi fish pond in the little park below the window.

The stack of paperwork I had to sign was more massive than I had to sign during a house purchase. Among the paperwork, there was an agreement that I was a guarantor of my mother's payments for the assisted living facility room and board. I was hesitant about signing this obligation as the cost hovered around $5,000 per month. On the other hand, I really liked this facility, and I was afraid they would reject her application if I did not sign it. So I signed it.

The payment schedule for the room and board worked like a typical apartment rental. My first payment covered the first and last month's costs, and I had to make a monthly payment by the 5th of each month. I agreed that I would notify the assisted living facility when my mother had three months of payments left in her savings account. The director of the facility did not explain why he needed a three-month notice. You will see later that the three months was a critical time frame as it gave me more options.

DID I MAKE A
BIG MISTAKE?

When I got home, I did an internet search on being a guarantor for payments and found statute 42 CFR 483.12(d)(2) of Federal Regulations on Public Health. I included a direct link to this law in Appendix at the end of this book. This statute was in the Admission Policy section. This statute says it is illegal to ask a family member to sign the paperwork as a guarantor.

Here is the exact quote from this document that starts at the bottom of page 50:

"(2) The facility must not require a third party guarantee of payment to the facility as a condition of admission or expedited admission, or continued stay in the facility. However, the facility may require an individual who has legal access to a resident's income or resources available to pay for facility care to sign a contract, with-

out incurring personal financial liability, to provide facility payment from the resident's income or resources."

I panicked that I had made a huge mistake and made an appointment to see an elder law attorney. If I could have had a do-over, I would have seen the lawyer first. The lawyer explained to me that the statute I found refers to nursing homes, but not assisted living facilities. Even though he would have recommended that I did not sign such paperwork, it was not illegal for the assisted living facility to ask me to sign this agreement.

For the next two years, I worried about what would happen after my mother ran out of money. I was afraid that the facility would tell me that my mother did not qualify for the nursing home even if she did. I feared that they would have a financial interest in keeping her as a resident instead of transferring her to a nursing home. Thankfully, my worries turned out to be groundless; the assisted living facility was accommodating throughout the process. Perhaps one of the reasons was that both the assisted living facility and the nursing home were part of the same company and the parent company was so they would not lose residents during the transfer from the assisted living to the nursing home.

Tip:

If you think you might need to transfer your loved one from an assisted living facility to a nursing home, keep in mind the financial interests of the companies involved as well as yours. If possible, try not to sign guarantor paperwork. Also, keep in mind that elder law attorneys specialize in answering these and similar questions.

LIFE IN AN ASSISTED LIVING FACILITY

My mother adjusted to her assisted living facility quickly. She liked her apartment. She enjoyed that she could stay in her studio as much as she wanted. Occasionally, she joined community activities but not often. Her primary interaction with other residents was during meal times. Sometimes, she ended up at a table with people she did not like, and the care coordinators moved her to a different table to be with people she liked better.

Most of all, I appreciated that they kept in touch with me via email, which was my preferred method of communication. I work in an environment that provides no privacy, so I was glad I did not have to use the phone to discuss these personal matters. I would use email to pass my mother's requests to them. Other times they would give me updates on her health, mood, or behavior. For example, when she refused to take showers or take medication, we would discuss options on how to handle the situation. They were always caring and responsive. It took a lot of worry out of my life, as I no longer worried about how she was doing while I was at work or why she did not answer the phone.

The next year and nine months went by quickly. I noticed my mother's dementia became more severe. Sometimes she thought I was her sister rather than her daughter. It was shocking the first time it happened. I did not know if I should try to change her mind or just go with the flow.

The assisted living staff helped me understand that people with dementia often picture themselves as their younger selves. So if my mother thought of herself as a middle-aged woman, how could another middle-aged woman be her daughter? I had to be her sister. It was only logical. The good news was that my mother forgot that she and her sister did not get along. She was happy to see me both when she thought I was her sister, and when she knew I was her daughter. The director of the assisted living told me that this is quite common. He said that his personal experience was very similar to mine.

His father thought he was his brother, with whom he did not get along all his life. When his father thought he, his son, was the brother, he treated "the brother" very affectionately.

THREE MONTHS WARNING

Three months before my mother's funds were exhausted, I notified the director of the assisted living facility. He told me that my mother now medically qualified for the nursing home level of assistance. She would meet the Medicaid financial requirement in three months when her total savings would fall below $2,000.

He informed me I had two choices. I could apply for Medicaid either before or after my mother moved into the nursing home. If I wanted to submit the Medicaid application before the transfer to the nursing home, I would need to wait until her savings dropped below the maximum required amount. Then, I would wait for her application to be approved, and as soon as she received Medicaid approval, she could move to the nursing home. The danger of this first option is that Medicaid would not complete the processing of the application in 30 days. In that case, the guarantor is responsible for the monthly costs of the assisted living facility since the balance left in her account would not cover the full amount of monthly fees.

The second option was to transfer her to the nursing home first, in which case, the nursing home required one month of private payment, roughly $10,000, due on the day of admission.. Once my mother was admitted, she would have to apply for Medicaid within 30 days of admission. If Medicaid application processing took over 30 days, the nursing home would require her to pay her part of the payment but would wait for Medicaid to pay the rest when her application was approved. The individual's portion of the fee is the person's total income minus the $72.80 allowance allowed for personal expenses. The danger of the second approach is that the application would be denied and the cost of the nursing home was approximately twice as much as the cost of the assisted living facility.

My thought process on the two options was that the chances of the denial were low, given her preliminary medical evaluation and the fact that she met the financial requirements. On the other hand, I thought the chances of the application processing taking more than 30 days were high, and that turned out to be true.

It was vital that we had this conversation three months before my mother's funds were completely exhausted. The three months of payments available in her savings meant that my mother had enough money to pay for either three months of assisted living or one month of assisted living and the 30-day private payment for the nursing home.

ORCHESTRATING THE TRANSFER FROM THE ASSISTED LIVING FACILITY TO THE NURSING HOME

I decided that it would be best to transfer mom to the nursing home with the 30-day private payment. Next, I had to calculate the timing of the transfer. The key was to make sure that the balance of my mother's bank account was under $2,000 after the 30-day private payment check cleared. My mother had just enough money to pay for one month in assisted living and to cover one-month of private payment in the nursing home. However, two years ago, during admission, she pre-paid the last month's rent, so she had to stay in the assisted living facility for one more month to spend down her savings.

One month later, I gave the assisted living facility a 30-day written notice that she was moving out. In my 30-day notice, I stated that I would be using the prepaid last-month deposit to pay for the final month of room and board. In the two years she was a resident at the assisted living facility, the price has increased twice, and I had to pay the difference be-tween the original last-month deposit and the cur-rent cost. At the same time, I notified the nursing home that my mother was interested in an open bed in the nursing home at the end of the next month.

For the timing of the transfer to work, the nursing home had to have an open bed in the second half of the final month in the assisted living residence. If there were no free beds, we would have to pay for an extra month of assisted living and wait for an open bed. The bed opened up eight days before the end of the month. For eight days, my mother paid for both places. On the positive side, it gave me eight days to clean the assisted living apartment and arrange for the removal of the old furniture. The removal of the old furniture from the assisted living apartment is the responsibility of the resident who is moving

KADY DASH

out.

ROOMS IN THE NURSING HOME

Medicaid only pays for non-private rooms. In the nursing home, I could not select a specific room, but I could state my mother's preference for the window side of the room. I have visited several facilities, and the accommodations in all of them were very similar. A cloth curtain separates the two living spaces in all double occupancy rooms. The window side of the room is typically slightly smaller but provides more privacy.

Two adjacent rooms share a bathroom. This arrangement means that four people share the toilet. Residents cannot store personal belongings in the lavatory since it does not have much room. The bathroom has a sink and a toilet; it has no shower. The shower room is on the same floor, and nurses help residents to use it twice a week.

The nursing home provides a bed, a dresser, and a wardrobe. Most of the furniture in my mother's assisted facility apartment had to be thrown out, but there was room to bring in a small table and two chairs.

The standard nursing home room does not include a telephone. If a resident wants to have a phone, they need to contact the phone company directly and have a technician come out and install the service for that specific resident. Each bed has a phone jack next to the bed. The phone company sends the bills to the resident at the nursing home address. After the first bill, I set up online payments through my mother's bank.

The rooms in the nursing home were not as nice as the rooms in the assisted living facility, but they were clean.

ADMISSION TO THE NURSING HOME

On the morning of the day my mother was to move to the nursing home, I stopped by the business office, paid the 30-day private pay amount, and signed the admission paperwork.

Tip:

Get a receipt for the payment. You will need to submit it with your Medicaid application.

The nursing home had quite a few forms but not as many as the assisted living facility. This time, I knew about the statute that said that nursing facilities could not require a personal financial guarantee as a condition of admitting a family member. The lawyer advised me not to sign anything that mentions either a guarantor or the term "responsible party." He told me that any time I signed a form, I should make a notation that the signature was made under the durable power of attorney. Following his instructions, under each signature I wrote *"POA for"* my-mother's-name.

I had a copy of the statute 42 CFR 483.12(d)(2) with me and was ready to pull it out if it became necessary. However, the nursing home had a copy of this statute in my paperwork, and I had to sign it to acknowledge that I had read it.

I also met with the head nurse to discuss my mother's special requirements. We discussed having her food chopped up so she can chew it with her dentures, her sleeping schedule, and her reluctance to take medications. We also discussed her habits, likes, and dislikes.

Per the recommendation of the assisted living director, I moved my mother to her new room first and then packed up all her belongings. I originally wanted to pack first and then move her and her stuff at the same time. However, the director said that in his experience that was more confusing and disruptive for someone with dementia. The assisted living staff provided me a cart for moving, and it took a few trips to move all her belongings.

On the evening after the move, my mother was confused and unsettled. Even though we had discussed the upcoming move for over a month, she kept saying this was not her home and that she did not want to stay in the new room. On the positive side, I liked how the nurses handled it by distracting her with questions about the things she liked to do. The next day she sounded much better, and a few days later she thought she had been in her new room for a long time.

OTHER PROVISIONS TO BE ON THE LOOKOUT FOR

When I had a consultation with the lawyer, he mentioned two other provisions that often appear in the nursing home agreements.

Eviction: It is illegal for the nursing home to authorize eviction for any reason other than the nursing home cannot meet the resident's needs, the resident's health has improved, the resident's presence is endangering other residents, or the nursing home is ceasing operations, or if a self-pay resident has not paid for care for at least fifteen days. If there are different situations listed in the agreement, con-

HOW TO FIND CARE FOR YOUR ELDERLY PARENT

sider striking them out.

Waivers: Any provision that waives the nursing home's liability for lost or stolen personal items is illegal. It is also unlawful for the nursing home to waive liability for the resident's health. If you see these provisions, request that they be removed.

RESIDENT PAYMENTS

My mother moved to the nursing home on April 22, and the 30-day private pay covered her expenses through May 22. The 30-day private payment did not cover the nine days from May 23 to May 31. This gap meant that there was an outstanding balance for May at the rate of $325 per day. Since I provided proof to the nursing home that the Medicaid application was submitted, the business manager said that the amount my mother was responsible for was the patient portion of the May payment. Medicaid would cover the costs over the individual's portion of the payment for the partial month after the application is approved.

The amount of patient responsibility varies from person to person based on their income. The amount owed is equal to all income (pension and social security) minus $72.80 monthly allowance. This payment is often referred to as "patient paid amount." I had to pay the 30-day private pay on April 22 and then the individual's portion of May's fees on May 1. This payment schedule was not clearly explained to me prior to admission. However, it is essential to understand how a partial month payment is handled when planning to spend down the amount of savings to under $2,000 as you don't want to go too much under $2,000 to ensure that individual has as much reserve funds as the rules allow.

Tip:

When calculating the amount owed to the nursing home, you are allowed to subtract payments automatically withdrawn for Medicare from the social security payment. This reduction is allowed only until your application is approved.

Once the Medicaid application was approved, the Commonwealth of Massachusetts Health and Human Services notified my mother that she no longer had to pay Medicare payments. Medicaid reimbursed my mother for the amounts withdrawn for Medicare starting with the date of eligibility. In my mother's case, the date of eligibility was the first day after the private pay period, May 23. The date of application approval was June 26, and I received the approval letter in early July. This time-line meant that Medicaid reimbursed her for nine days in May and the months of June and July.

Remember that a person can keep only $72.80 every month regardless of their income. The fixed allowance amount meant that the payments due to the nursing home had to increase by the amount previously withdrawn to pay for Medicare.

The Medicaid reimbursement was automatically deposited into my mother's bank account. I had to forward that amount to the nursing home as the room and board due for the previous two months and nine days. The nursing home was owed this amount because the payments to the nursing home, before the Medicaid application was approved, were reduced by the amount of Medicare payments.

INITIAL MEDICAID APPLICATION

The Medicaid application form is available online for each state. The full name of the form is "Application for Health Coverage for Seniors and People Needing Long-Term-Care Services." A link to the application is available in the Appendix.

The application is about 20 pages long, and I thought some terminology was ambiguous. I imagined how my mother (or any elderly person) would struggle to complete this application on her own. I felt it would be difficult for her, as it requires good organization skills, good memory, and attention to detail.

When I saw the elder law attorney, he said that he provides a service of completing the Medicaid application, but the cost for this service is several thousand dollars. He typically gets involved when there are reasons to think that denial is likely due to some financial transactions. He also mentioned that there are businesses where non-lawyers help people complete the application, and because they are not lawyers, the price of the service is less. Overall, he told me to examine her financial records and if there were no transactions over $1,000 in the last five years he thought the application process should be relatively smooth and I should be able to handle it on my own.

The Medicaid application mostly identifies a person's financial situation. The form asks for the following supporting documents: proof of income, tax returns for the last three years, statements from banks and other financial institutions for the previous 60 months (5 years), and proof of citizenship/legal immigration status. If the application is being submitted by a family member with power of attorney, they must also include the power of attorney paperwork.

I only had access to eighteen months of bank statements through on-line access. The nursing home business manager told me to submit what I had, and if what I sent was not sufficient, I would get a request for additional information. She told me that the Medicaid office would give me 30 days to provide supplemental materials.

The eighteen months of bank records turned out to be sufficient. However, the request for additional information I received included requests for information going back as far as eight years, six years, and three years. On the positive side, the caseworker demanded information about specific transactions, not the entire history going that far back. I will describe the details of what the caseworker wanted in a later chapter.

APPLICATION QUESTIONS CLARIFICATIONS

The business manager of the nursing home told me I could ask her questions if I needed help with the Medicaid application forms. I took advantage of her offer by sending her a draft of the application with questions on the areas I found confusing. Below are the clarifications I needed to be confident I was providing the right information.

Question 1: Address/Mailing address. Is it to okay to specify my home address as a mailing address?

The answer to this question was "Yes", however mailings did not work the way I expected.

I wanted all correspondence regarding the appli-

HOW TO FIND CARE FOR YOUR ELDERLY PARENT

cation, and any follow-up questions mailed to my home address, not to my mother's nursing home address. The form provided two sections for address: address and mailing address. I specified my mother's address in the nursing home as the address and my address as the mailing address. My expectation was that all paperwork would come to me, and that my mother would not be getting any mail during the application process. However, the Medicaid caseworker sent paperwork to both addresses, including the denial letter. If that letter had reached my mother, she would have been very confused, upset, and concerned. Luckily, I had arranged for the nursing home to forward my mother's mail to my home address so I could pay her bills in a timely matter. Therefore, the copy of the denial letter from Medicaid sent to my mother was, thankfully, also forwarded to me. Thank God for that, the last thing I needed was to have her panic about the denial without knowing what to do. I will cover the application denial and how I handled it later in the book.

Tip:

If you are taking care of the bills for your parent, consider making a mail forwarding arrangement with the nursing home.

Question 16: DISABILITY. Do you have a disability (including a disabling mental health condition) that has lasted or expected to last for at least 12 months?

It was not clear to me if dementia was a disability, and if the answer to this question should be "Yes." The nursing home business manager told me that dementia is not considered a disability. However, she also told me I could answer this question "Yes" if I wanted and specify "dementia."

Question 17: Do you need reasonable accommodations because of a disability?

This item was the only place on the application where I could note down what type of special accommodations my mother required because of her dementia (such as administration of medication, help with showers, special food preparation, and so on). Since I answered "Yes" to question 16, I could write the required accommodations in this item. As I learned later, this information on the application form was unnecessary because Medicaid sent a nurse to assess my mom's clinical condition. The nurse collected all the required information by examining my mother and talking to the head nurse responsible for my mother's care.

Question 27: Other income. Social Security benefit.

It was not clear to me if the number entered on the form should be the amount before or after Medicare Plan B payment was deducted from the Social Security benefit. The clarification I got was that this amount should be the amount of the Social Security benefit *after* subtracting the Medicare Plan B payment.

This clarification was correct but it was not a complete answer. Medicare payments could be deducted from the Social Security for the purpose of calculating income only until the Medicaid application approval. When the Medicaid application was approved, Medicare Plan B payments were no longer withdrawn from the monthly Social Security pension deposits. My mother's income increased by the amount previously paid to Medicare. However, Medicaid rules allow a person to keep only $72.80 each month, so the increase in income also resulted in an increase of the amount owed to the nursing home by the amount previously paid for Medicare Plan B.

Step 4: Previous Medical Bills. Do you have bills for medical services you got in the three months before the month we got your application?

I answered "No" because at the time of my mother's transfer to the nursing home she had no outstanding bills. This was the wrong answer because the question includes the period up to the application *approval* which is not the same as "when we got your application." In the two months that my mother's application was being processed, she accumulated medical bills, and Medicaid would have paid for some of these bills if the answer was "Yes."

Note that I said "some" rather than "all" bills. The bills my mother received during the first month (the period when her boarding expenses were covered by the private payment) were not eligible for re-reimbursement because, during that month, she did not qualify financially. At the start of that month, she had $12,000 in her savings account, and the amount went down to $2,000 only after she made a payment to the nursing home.

The Medicaid caseworker changed the answer to "Yes" while processing the paperwork; I did not have to resubmit the application to make this change. I will come back to this topic when I describe the phone call with the caseworker after the application denial when she told me the right answer to this question.

Step 5 Question 1: Bank accounts. Current balance

and balance on admission date.

My mother's savings account balance was several hundred dollars over the required amount. My question was if I could pay this extra amount to the nursing home on the day of admission. The answer was "Yes."

To be eligible for Medicaid, the current balance of all savings must be under $2,000. However, suppose your loved one's balance is over the $2,000 amount. In this case, you can do what they call a "spend-down" payment by making an extra payment to the nursing home over the minimum amount you owe. Suppose the 30-day private pay is $10,000, and after that payment your loved one has $3,000 left in their savings account. You can make a payment of $11,000 to bring you down to the $2,000 amount. So, in this case, the application will show $2,000 as the current balance and $13,000 as the balance on the admission date. If you don't make an extra spend-down payment and leave the extra money in the parent's account, the Medicaid application will be denied because the balance is larger than the allowed maximum.

Step 5: Assets. Do you have bank accounts, certificates of deposits, checking, savings, credit union, NOW, market, and personal needs allowance (PNA account)? You must provide information about both opened and closed accounts. Provide proof

for the past 60 months.

I had easy access to 18 months worth of statements rather than the 60 months that the application required. I asked the nursing home business manager if I should send a request to the bank to provide the additional statements. She told me to submit what I had and wait to see what other information the Medicaid office requested. This way, I had to contact the bank only once in case the Medicaid caseworker asked me for something that was not included in my first request.

Step 5 Question 9: Prepaid burial plans.

If the "extra" amount in savings is several thousand dollars, you may purchase a prepaid burial plan. Medicaid allows this expense and does not count it towards the $2,000 savings maximum amount. The "extra" amount in my mother's account was too small to investigate this option.

Step 6: Medicare coverage. Start dates for Medicare Part A and Medicare Plan D.

I did not have this information. The manager said it was okay to make my best guess and make a note that I am not sure of the actual start date.

Step 7: Personal-care-attendant Services and cor-

responding Supplement C: Personal-care attendant

If your loved one is in the nursing home, personal-care-attendant services do not apply. The services in Step 7 cover a person living at home and using personal-care-attendant services.

Supplement A: Long-term care.

Complete this supplement when a long-term nursing home is needed.

Supplement A Question 18: Tax returns.

This form requires you to submit your parent's last two years of U.S. income tax returns. If you do not have copies, you need to fill out and sign IRS form 4506. The only exception is if a person's income is below the filing limit. In that case, proof of income for those two years is sufficient.

Authorized Representative Designation form.

There are three options for selecting a representative. The person applying for Medicaid can enlist someone else to help them complete the form and respond to follow-up questions from the Medicaid caseworker.

Option 1: If the applicant (your parent) can sign, they need to sign Section 1 Part 1 of the form. In this case, Section 1 Part 2 of the form must be completed and signed by the representative.

Option 2: If you are the representative, but do not have power of attorney, and your parent can no longer sign a form, use Section 2 representative.

Option 3: If the representative is appointed by law, such as a power of attorney, use Section 3 representative. The application package must also include a copy of the power of attorney paperwork.

Note: If you use Section 2 or Section 3 representative, the applicant does not need to sign the application.

I used Section 3 representative designation acting as a power of attorney for my mother.

TIMELINE FOR PROCESSING THE MEDICAID APPLICATION

The nursing home required me to provide them a copy of the application and proof that I had mailed it within 30 days of admission (i.e., during the 30-day private pay period). My mother transferred to the nursing home on April 22. I sent the Medicaid application on May 1, which was the day I saw the 30-day private pay check had cleared through the bank. I waited for the check to clear so I could include the latest bank statement that showed the amount of savings under $2,000. I printed statements from the on-line access to the bank account. The proof of mailing was the receipt from the post office with the tracking number. I also

attached the information from USPS online tracking, which showed when the package was delivered.

Medicaid processed the application on May 9 based
on the date of the letter requesting additional information. The Medicaid office sent the package by
regular mail, and I received it on May 20. The letter
gave me a deadline of June 9 for providing the information to them, which was 30 days from the date
they processed the application. However, I received
this letter 11 days later, so the letter gave me only
three weeks to get the information. Financial institutions were not able to process the paperwork and
send it back to me in this time frame.

The short deadline caused me a tremendous
amount of stress. Nobody told me that the first 30-
day deadline is not a hard deadline, and it is one of
the reasons I am writing this book. I want to clarify
the process for caregivers so you can avoid the stress
and sleepless nights I went through. As you will see
in the later chapters, after the initial 30-day deadline and denial, the Medicaid office gave me another
30 days to complete gathering the information.

REQUEST FOR ADDITIONAL INFORMATION

The Medicaid office has its own sources of information about each applicant. The letter requested supplemental details about items that I did not include in the application package. The accounts that the Medicaid office was interested in were closed over five years ago, and the application stated that I needed to include information going back five years. The caseworker asked for the statements that covered the previous calendar year from a mutual fund company where my mother had an IRA account that was closed eight years ago. She also wanted a detailed history of the certificates of deposit (listed by CD account numbers) that included one CD that was cashed six years ago. The other CDs were closed and transferred to my mother's checking account two years ago and were used to pay for the assisted living facility. The caseworker wanted to see the history of the money movement, i.e., withdrawals from CDs, where the money was transferred to, and how the money was used.

To complicate things, the caseworker referred to CDs by the name of a bank that no longer exists. My mother's old bank was acquired several years ago by another bank. However, I had to prove that my mother had an account with only one bank, not two.

Besides asking about the accounts mentioned above, the Medicaid caseworker asked me to annotate each deposit and withdrawal over $1,000 on the checking account statements I already provided. The caseworker was also interested in seeing copies of all checks with a value of over $1,000. The information about deposits may uncover hidden sources of income; checks might help her see if the recipient is transferring money to other people rather than using it for their own expenses.

Finally, the letter included a request for additional information related to the nursing home. The request contained a number of acronyms and form names which were not familiar to me. The letter said: *"Provide permission to share, a PNA state-*

HOW TO FIND CARE FOR YOUR ELDERLY PARENT

ment, and a private pay statement showing what has been paid to date and the date range covered. Provide SC-1 form and Nursing Facility screening notification." I contacted the business manager at the nursing home, and she told me she would fax PSI, SC-1, Screening Notification from Elder Services, PNA, and Payment letter directly to the caseworker.

It took a little research to understand what all these abbreviations stand for. Links to the referenced forms are available in the Appendix. Briefly, the acronyms are:

PSI is permission to share form. It is a HIPAA form signed during admission to the nursing home.

SC-1 is a status change form. This form is a notification of admission form signed during admission to the nursing home.

Screening Notification from Elder Services is the report generated after the clinical assessment of the resident.

The PNA form shows whether a resident maintains a personal needs account with the nursing facility. Some residents have their allowance deposited into these accounts, so they have access to petty cash. The balance of this account is added to the applicant's other savings. Together, the balance of all savings must be below $2,000.

Tip:

When communicating with Medicaid, always include the first page of the letter to which you are responding. The first page contains the name of the applicant, the unique ID of the applicant, the number of the notice, and the name of the caseworker assigned to the case.

DIFFICULTIES GETTING INFORMATION AS THE POWER OF ATTORNEY

The information I needed to collect fell into two categories: the information I could quickly get myself online or find in my mother's records; and the paperwork that required a financial institution to do research for me. I found the history of the bank merger on the bank's website. The merger history proved that the CDs from two different banks were, in fact, the same thing as the account numbers were the same and only the bank name had changed. I could also print copies of all checks over $1,000, as they were all payments made to the assisted living facility in the last two years. I sent the first batch of information to Medicaid well within the June 9 deadline.

The information that required research by financial institutions would prove to be very difficult. I had to deal with two different financial companies. One of them did not recognize my power of attorney paperwork at all; the second one took an extra week to approve it, which in turn pushed me a week over the June 9 Medicaid deadline.

Tip:

> *Financial institutions charge for researching information about your account. This fee is waived if a requester submits a form called "Financial Information Request" from the Medicaid website (A link to this form is available in the Appendix). When you submit this form, the bank is obligated to provide this information, free of charge, within two weeks of the form submission. Be aware that, in my case, it took longer than two weeks because of the extra time required to approve my power of attorney document. Two weeks is just a guideline.*

As mentioned earlier, I needed information from a mutual fund where my mother had an IRA. My name was not on that account as it was opened and closed while my mother did not need help to handle her finances. I also needed historical information for security deposits from the bank where my mother had her CDs. My mom had added my name as a second person on the checking account and CDs so I could pay bills on her behalf.

WHEN A POWER OF ATTORNEY HAS NO POWER

For the mutual fund, I found that my mother saved a statement from eight years ago, showing that the balance went to zero that year. The Medicaid caseworker requested the statements from last year showing the current balance, not a statement from eight years ago. So my goal was to get a letter from the mutual fund stating the account was closed eight years ago, and the balance remained zero since then. I called the mutual fund company to find out what paperwork I should send them to get this confirmation. The mutual fund representative said they could not provide me any information even if I sent them my power of attorney paperwork along with the request. The representative told me that my mother would need to make me a limited agent for the account before they would speak to me.

I printed the limited agent form, had my mother sign it and overnighted the package to them. I also included a copy of the power of attorney document, a letter from her doctor confirming she has dementia, and the last statement from eight years. The next communication from the mutual fund company was that this paperwork was not valid because they cannot make a limited agent for a closed account.

I asked if they could confirm that the account was closed eight years ago if my mother wrote a letter requesting this confirmation. They said "OK," and I had my mother sign this new request and I overnighted the second package to them. When they received that package, they said they couldn't honor it because along with the copy of a power of attorney, I included a letter from my mother's doctor that stated she had dementia. I thought this letter would help me get results quickly. Unfortunately, it turned out to have the opposite effect. They told me in order to make her request valid; I would need a letter from a doctor that stated that my mother does have dementia.

When I told them that this would not be possible, they said that the next option I had was to send them the original power of attorney paperwork because they don't know if the copy I sent them had been modified from the original. I needed the original for other matters I had to do on behalf of my mother. Besides, I was afraid that if the post office lost the package, it would leave me with no original at all.

The mutual fund representative's next suggestion was to go to my bank and request they validate a copy of the power of attorney paperwork with a medallion signature guarantee. I went to my bank where they told me they don't provide medallion signature guarantees for legal paperwork. They told me they have no way of knowing if the original paperwork I brought with me is, in fact, the original. They were apologetic but firm that this is not their area of expertise and they could not help me.

The exchange with the mutual fund company exasperated me. I was not asking for any information that I did not already have. I was not trying to take over an account with money. They refused to help me because the procedure was more important than the intent. They called it "protecting their client." I even offered them to send the information directly to the Medicaid office rather than to me, but they still said they could not do it.

By June 6, I had nothing but the email communications saying that they cannot do anything for me. Because I have my money invested with the same mutual fund company, I could communicate with them via their secure mail. Email communication at least gave me a paper trail of our conversations, which I would not have had if I only talked to them on the phone. I submitted these emails along with the eight-year-old statement with a zero balance to Medicaid. The line I highlighted was the line where the mutual fund representative stated that he could not give me limited agent power over a closed account. Since he referred to a closed account, he confirmed that the account was closed. Fortunately, Medicaid accepted this combination of information, and I could satisfy their request for additional information about this account.

Tip:

If possible, communicate via email rather than the phone because emails leave an electronic trail that you might be able to use as a confirmation. Better yet, have your parents collect the information about all accounts, including the closed ones, while they still can.

MISSING THE DEADLINE

My mother's bank, at least, did not reject my power of attorney outright. The bank took an extra week validating my power of attorney paperwork. In the past, they had seen the original paperwork in person. I visited the bank office along with my mother several times before she moved to the assisted living facility. Perhaps this was the reason they, at least, eventually approved the paperwork. The bank received the form on May 22, but on June 7, when I checked the status of my request, they said I would receive the response in a week. I notified the Medicaid caseworker of the delay because of the time it took to approve the power of attorney paperwork and requested a one-week extension. The bank paperwork arrived a week later. I sent the package using overnight mail, and the Medicaid office signed for it

HOW TO FIND CARE FOR YOUR ELDERLY PARENT

on June 17.

THE DENIAL

June 17 was past June 9 deadline. The extension I had requested was not granted, and I received a denial letter dated June 18. The letter stated that the application was denied because the Medicaid office had not received the additional information they requested. The denial letter listed the account numbers for each CD. The CD history was the information they had received on June 17. However, the critical positive piece of information in the denial letter was that this was not the final denial. The letter said that if I could supply the missing information within 30 days from the day they generated the denial letter (i.e., by July 17) the application would be automatically re-submitted with a new date.

I did not know what the correct next step was. Should I resubmit the CD information again, or should I wait and see if what I had sent would be enough? I also did not know the ramifications of the application date change. Since the one-month private pay ended on May 22, who would be responsible for the June payment to the nursing home? I also received two medical bills in the mail and was not sure what to do about them.

After a sleepless night, I called the Medicaid office. As expected, I did not get a person; I got an answering machine. I left a message explaining that I had mailed the missing information and tracking showed that the letter had been delivered. I got a call back in about two hours. The caseworker assigned to handle my mother's case told me that she had received the letter and that that everything looked OK, but she needed two additional pieces of information. She had sent a new letter dated June 20 listing the details she wanted to see. At the time of our telephone conversation, I had not yet received this letter.

She told me she wanted more information about a check for several hundred dollars deposited in May 2018. This check was a refund of the safety deposit from my mother's old apartment. I suppose, to the examiner it could have looked like an undisclosed source of income. For some reason, the bank records only showed the back of the check, not the front, which showed who issued the check. Fortunately, I had made a copy of the check before depositing it.

The second piece of information she wanted explained was a $2,000 deposit in 2016. She said that she could not find the source for this deposit, which turned out to be an oversight on her part. This withdrawal was on the history of one of the CDs I had provided to the Medicaid office. As my mother rolled over that CD, she withdrew $2,000. The CD withdrawal had a matching deposit into her savings account on the same day. I was able to highlight these two transactions in my response.

I asked the caseworker about the ramifications of the date change of the application. She explained that the change in the application date was not significant, because Medicaid would pay the bills up to three months prior to the application approval. She confirmed she would update the portion of the application where I marked that there were no outstanding bills before application submission.

The caseworker on the phone was pleasant, patient, and helpful. Given the stressful situation, she made me feel less stressed. I said that I would provide additional information for both issues as soon as possible. She also said I could fax information rather than mail it.

I found the relevant info for both questions and faxed the explanations to the phone number included in the letter. Sending a fax from my home

HOW TO FIND CARE FOR YOUR ELDERLY PARENT

machine does not give me an explicit confirmation that the fax successfully reached the recipient. The fax log only shows that the fax was sent successfully. I decided to mail the same information via over-night mail in order to have a signature confirmation that the package was delivered before the July 17 deadline.

MEDICAL ASSESSMENT

The financial and the clinical evaluation happens at the same time. While the Medicaid application was being processed, I received a phone call from the Elder Services nurse who performed my mother's evaluation under regulations 130 CMR 456 (Long-term care services) and 130 CMR 408 (Adult foster care). She informed me that my mother qualified for the services. A few days later, I received an official letter confirming her clinical eligibility. This letter arrived 19 days before the first Medicaid deadline.

Links to 130 CMR 456 and 130 CMR 408 regulations are available in the Appendix. These regulations list the clinical requirements that an individual must meet in order to qualify for Medicaid services.

THE APPROVAL

The first sign that the application was approved was not the approval letter from Medicaid but a letter from the Department of Health and Human Services stating that my mother qualified for a discount on Medicare Part D drug plan.

On July 8, I received the letter that my mother would be eligible for standard Medicaid benefits. The eligibility began May 23, which was the first day after the 30-day private pay period ended. The letter also stated her new patient paid amount. Once my mother was approved for Medicaid, Medicare stopped deducting Medicare payments from her Social Security. The patient paid amount was increased by the amount she previously paid for Medicare. The letter stated that Medicaid would reimburse the Medicare payments she had paid for May, June, and July, and these reimbursements should be redirected to the nursing home. The letter noted that the refunds would reach her in a few months. In a few weeks, I received another letter stating that the reimbursement would be deposited into my mother's account on August 8. However, the deposits were made earlier than promised: Medicare Plan D amount was deposited on July 11 and Medicare reimbursement on July 25.

ANNUAL RE-CERTIFICATIONS

What is the Medicaid process after the initial approval? The nursing home business manager told me that, annually, typically on the anniversary date of approval, Medicaid will send eligibility review forms to the nursing home facility and the individual. From the individual, they require financial records for the previous two months and the current stubs for any pension payments. From the facility, they require clinical re-evaluation.

LIFELINE PROGRAM

Once the Medicaid application is approved, the person will qualify for a Lifeline program that provides discounted telephone services for low-income individuals. The charges vary slightly from state to state.

The Commonwealth of Massachusetts rates are:

Voice Lifeline Flat Rate Unlimited - $8.10

Voice Lifeline Measured Service - $1.16

Broadband (internet) - $9.25 monthly discount

The actual bills were around $3 per month after taxes.

Tip:

The Lifeline program changed its application form in the last year or two. If you use an old form it will be rejected. I initially used the wrong application. I searched online and happened to find the old form first. When the application was rejected by the phone company, the reason was not clear. I had to call the phone company to figure out what I did incorrectly. They explained that Lifeline is a federal government program, and it requires that you use the latest form. The current form is FCC FORM 5629 (look in the upper left corner). A link to the Lifeline program information for all US states and a link to the application itself is available in the Appendix. However, make sure that you use the most recent form, which may be different.

SENIOR CARE OPTIONS PLANS

Another program available to a person who is approved for Medicaid is a Senior Care Option medical plan. Senior care option programs are available to people 65 or older who qualify for both Medicare and Medicaid. These plans provide a member with more coverage than Medicare and Medicaid alone. For example, these policies pay for diabetic shoes, complete dentures, and glasses, whereas Medicaid and Medicare do not. There are no additional charges to join the plan, and there are no co-pays for doctor visits. In addition, members of this program receive $100 every three months on a card that can be used at CVS, Walgreens, or Rite Aid. The money on the card can be spent only on pre-approved items such as cold medications, bandages, antibiotic ointments, or dental care. The rules also include a long list of items

HOW TO FIND CARE FOR YOUR ELDERLY PARENT

that are not eligible, such as hearing aid batteries, deodorants, dry skin remedies, shampoos, foot insoles, and much more.

Massachusetts has several Senior Care Option plans offered by different providers. However, a nursing home may be contracted to work with a particular program. My mother's nursing home has a contract with Senior Whole Health. So even though in theory, Massachusetts offered multiple options, I did not have a choice of a provider.

Be aware that enrolling in a Senior Care Options plan will dis-enroll the person from the previous Medicare Prescription Plan D plan. The disenrollment letter reached me before the letter stating that my mother had Medicare Prescription Plan D coverage with Senior Care Option as provider and I was confused and concerned for one day that she had no coverage at all until I got a clarification.

INTERVIEW QUESTIONS

T he next several chapters of the book contain the questions to ask the staff of assisted living facilities and nursing homes during your initial evaluation visits. I have a separate set of chapters for assisted living facilities and nursing homes. The services each facility provides are different enough that the important questions for each are different. I also include the answers that I received as a point of reference for comparison when you do your own interviews. I found how each facility handled a long list of questions as revealing as the answers themselves. The facilities I liked most patiently answered all my questions, did not push me towards an immediate decision and did not sound like salespeople.

When I visited assisted living facilities, I organized

my questions using a spreadsheet. The questions were in the left-most column and each facility had answers in a separate column. This way, it was easy to compare the answers I received from different facilities. If you would like a copy of the spreadsheet please refer to the Conclusion chapter.

QUESTIONS TO ASK ASSISTED LIVING FACILITIES

*Questions about the costs
in assisted living facility*

What is the occupancy fee? Are there different rooms at different prices?

Some facilities charge residents based on the size of the room. Others charged solely based on the number of rooms (one-bedroom, two-bedroom, or studio) regardless of the differences in size.

What are the personal care fees?

In my mother's assisted living facility, a few hours of personal care were included as part of the base fee. If she needed more personal care, the charge was $1 per minute. How much personal care she needed each month varied, there were months when she did not get charged any additional fee and months where she was charged two hundred or three hundred dollars.

Is a phone line provided? Is there a phone fee?

In the beginning, the assisted living facility charged my mother a $25 fee each month. Then, after a fee increase, this expense was included in the occupancy fee. I considered getting a cheap pre-paid cell phone, but she was not able to learn how to use it. This is typical for people with dementia, they cannot retain new information. My mother did not recognize a cell phone as a phone that could be used to make and receive phone calls. When the cell phone rang she kept looking for an object that looked like a phone that she remembered. How to answer the phone and the need to charge it every day was too complicated as well.

Is cable TV provided? Is there a fee for cable service?

In my mother's facility, the TV set was provided, as well as the cable service. The fee was included in the occupancy fee. Even though my mother never watched TV (prior and after moving to assisted living), they still charged her for the cable service. This fee was not optional and not negotiable.

Does the assisted living facility do laundry? How much does it cost?

The laundry fee was determined by weight. The family of the resident had the option to do laundry themselves. I did most of the laundry myself. Sometimes the staff felt something needed to get washed right away and then they added a laundry fee to the monthly bill.

Tip:

Put labels on clothing and other items that might go into the assisted living laundry. I used a permanent marker to write my mom's name or her initials on things. The tags will prevent items from getting mixed up with someone else's stuff. What items to label? I would say whatever is washable should have a tag. One of my mother's blankets got lost in the laundry, so I put labels on everything, including blankets. If you are wondering what happened with the lost comforter... It was never found, but the facility replaced the missing blanket with a similar one the day I reported it.

Are linens provided?

In my mother's facility, linens, and towels were provided as part of the occupancy fee. The linens were laundered once a week. If a resident had an accident, the laundry was done the same day. For example, my mother enjoyed sucking on a chocolate bar as she fell asleep, so chocolate stains often covered her pillowcase and required more frequent changes. The facility did not charge an extra fee for extra linens washes.

What other supplies are provided?

My mother's assisted living provided toilet paper, shampoo, and soap.

Tip:

To avoid surprises, ask what the occupancy fee does not cover.

Is transportation provided to doctor appointments, shopping?

In our case, transportation to doctors was the family responsibility. However, my mother began using the doctor associated with the facility, so I never had to take her to medical appointments. The facility organized weekly shopping trips, but my mother did not take part in them as I purchased everything that she needed.

Is there a community fee?

A community fee is a one-time entrance fee. The admission's coordinator told me it covered the nurse visit to my mother's home for a mandatory medical evaluation. Not all facilities sent a nurse for a visit; some facilities required me to bring my mother in for evaluation instead which was more stressful for her.

Is there a 30-day termination notice?

The resident must give a 30-day notice that they are leaving the facility. This applies when the resident moves to either a nursing home or to a different facility. I was told that this payment would be collected even when the resident dies; the resident will still be responsible for one extra month of room and board.

Is there a prepaid final month fee?

This fee covers the last occupancy payment. It works in tandem with a 30-day termination notice and must be paid in advance during admission. Since my mother was transferred to the nursing home, we used this prepaid amount to cover her last month's occupancy fee in the assisted living facility.

Does the assisted living facility require a family member to be a guarantor for the payments?

This guarantee is illegal for nursing homes but not unlawful for assisted living facilities. If this language exists in the assisted living facility agreement, ask if it is mandatory.

Is there a non-refundable deposit to hold the room?

This deposit covers the period after you select the room and the start of the residency. For me, it was eight days and the amount of the fee was $1,000. The room deposit was credited towards the first-month payment.

Does this facility accept Medicare?

Medicare does not pay for room and board, but it does pay for a portion of medicine, doctor visits, and physical therapy. Therefore, you want to make sure that the facility accepts Medicare as all residents will have medical expenses.

Does this facility accept Medicaid?

Medicaid does not cover assisted living. However, if there is a nursing home associated with the same facility, then this question is relevant because Medicaid does cover nursing home expenses.

What happens when the resident runs out of money?

Some facilities have other means of providing financial assistance to residents (private funds, state funds). If the facility does not have financial assistance, they should explain the option of moving to the nursing home and applying for Medicaid for those residents that meet the Medicaid requirements. If the staff is knowledgeable, they should be able to explain both the medical and financial aspects of who can qualify for the assistance.

If the person you are talking to does not give you the answer to the previous question, then explicitly ask if there is a financial support program for low-income residents. Find out what income qualifies as low income. Ask if there is a waiting list for these subsidized rooms.

Ask about annual price increases.

Request a price quote not only for the current year but for the previous year and the year before that for comparison. Expect the cost to increase each year. In my mother's facility, the cost increase was approximately 5% a year.

What happens if a resident's condition gets worse, and they need memory care?

It is helpful to know if there is a memory facility in the same building. Memory care is long-term care designed to meet the needs of a person with Alzheimer's disease, dementia, or other types of memory problems. Memory care facilities have therapeutic programs aimed at memory impaired, they are often color-coded to help residents find their way around the facility, and typically provide more security to prevent residents from wandering away and getting lost.

Is there a dementia fee? What is the amount of this fee?

The extra charge for memory care units in my mother's facility was $550 a month. The nurse evaluation was that my mother did not need memory care at this time. My impression was that this care was for the people who wandered away, as a memory unit section was a locked section.

*Questions about selecting
a room in an assisted
living facility*

Is there a choice of rooms? Ask to see the apartments. Ask for permission to take photos.

I saw at least one room in each facility I visited. I asked to take photos and, in most cases, was permitted to take pictures as long as they did not include any residents. These photographs were helpful for me to remember and compare different facilities. I also showed them to my mother, so that she could feel part of the decision making. For the facility I have selected, I had a choice of three studio apartments. One apartment was larger with a view onto a parking lot. One was across from the dining room, and I thought it would be noisy. The third apartment was smaller but had a beautiful view from the window. I selected the smaller room with the nicest view.

Tip:

Bring a measuring tape so that you can measure walls. Measurements will be helpful when you are figuring out what furniture to bring and what will fit and will not fit in the room.

What furniture is provided?

The room included a bed, a dresser, a nightstand with a lamp, and a chair. My mother wanted to bring her own bed, so I asked for the bed provided by the facility to be removed. We were able to move in two more dressers, a table, and a few armchairs.

Does the room have a microwave?

The studio apartment had a small kitchen that included a microwave and a small refrigerator. My mother never had a microwave before and, so, she never fully learned how to use it. She could not remember my instructions to heat things only for 1 minute. Every week, I would find the microwave dirty from explosions of whatever she was trying to warm up. Eventually, I unplugged the microwave because it felt dangerous for her to continue using it.

Can a resident eat in their room if they wish?

This practice was discouraged from being used regularly. Taking left-overs back to the room was not a problem.

Will a meal be brought to the room on request by the resident?

The staff brought lunches and dinners to a resident's room if they were not feeling well. However, if the resident was feeling fine, they were expected to eat in the common dining room.

General questions about the assisted living facility

What type of units does this facility have: independent livings, assisted living, memory care, skilled nursing?

The facility I selected had assisted living and memory care in one building, and memory care and skilled nursing in the nursing home connected to it.

Check if there is a pleasant area outside. Are the residents allowed to spend time outside on their own?

My mother did not go outside on her own. However, when I visited, we often went for a walk and it was nice to have a pleasant area where we could walk safely and had something to look at (e.g., fish pond, bird feeders, flowers).

How many residents are in the facility? How many men, how many women, what is their average age?

How many staff members are in the facility during the day, evening, and on weekends?

How are the new attendants trained? Do they go through background checks?

Is there a nurse on staff?

The attendants who take care of the residents in the assisted living facility do not have medical training, they are not nurses. In addition to attendants, in my mother's facility, there was always one nurse on-premises. She was one of my primary contacts, and we exchanged emails at least once a week.

Is there a regular doctor who visits the residents? How often is he or she on the premises?

In the mother's facility, the doctor came once a week, but the exact time of his visits was not known week to week. I found this unpredictability a little frustrating because my mother would always ask me when he would come, and I could not tell her. However, I spoke with him on the phone several times and found him helpful and responsive.

Is there a podiatrist to help residents with nail cutting?

I asked my mother about nail cutting a few times, and she told me everything was fine. Then a few months later, I asked her to show me her toenails, and I saw that her nails were so long that they were curling. I made an appointment with a podiatrist for her, and he took care of her toenails. My mother hates doctors, but she told me she liked this doctor and how he trimmed her toenails!

Tip:

Trust but verify. I should have asked to see my mom's toenails rather than just asking her about them.

Is there a hair salon on the premises? How much does it cost?

The assisted living facility had a hair salon open once a week, and the residents could get their hair cut on a schedule of their preference. The haircuts were $25, and the amount was added to the monthly bill.

Is there a library?

The assisted living facility had an extensive library. My mother enjoyed reading and would bring dozens of books into her apartment every week. When I visited, we went through the books she accumulated in her room, and I would take the ones she said she was done with back to the library. The extensive collection of books that migrated to her apartment was never brought up to me as an issue.

What activities are provided for the residents? Are the residents required to take part in activities if they don't wish to participate?

If your parent is a person who does not like to socialize, make sure the assisted living facility will not force them to take part in activities if they don't want to do so. Some facilities were more receptive to free will, whereas others felt socializing was important for residents' welfare. Since you know your parents best, make sure that there is a good fit in this area, as they will need to deal with this aspect every day.

Can the kitchen handle special food prep, for example, chopping food for every meal for someone with dentures?

Ask to look at the weekly menu. See if there is a good variety of foods for each meal, and, in general, during the week.

What are the assisted living alcohol policies?

If your loved one enjoys a glass of wine with dinner ask about alcohol policies. The foremost concern of assisted living facilities is to keep their residents safe. Seniors can be vulnerable to problems from alcohol even when they consume only modest amounts. Assisted living communities have widely varying alcohol policies. Some are totally dry, some allow residents to have wine in the room, others allow alcohol consumption with meals. My mother's facility did not allow alcohol in premises.

Do residents have a choice at what time they have breakfast, lunch and dinner?

In my mother's facility, the answer I got during the interview was "No." The residents' breakfast was 8 to 9, lunch 12 to 1, and dinner 5 to 6. However, my mother often went to the dining room on her own schedule say at 11:00 and 4:00, and they accommodated her unusual hours and never complained to me.

Are there visiting hours?

The assisted living facility did not have visiting hours. Guests were welcomed at any time. However, the doors were locked at 8 pm and visitors who came after 8 pm had to buzz in.

Are overnight guests allowed?

Some facilities permit overnight guests staying in the resident's apartment. Some facilities have guest rooms available for rent for out of town guests. In addition, guests can join residents during a meal for a fee. At my mother's facility the guest meal fee was $25.

Is there a bedtime curfew?

I was not told about any evening curfew. My mother went to bed early, so this topic did not come up in conversations. However, I had to speak to the staff about the morning schedule. My mother liked to sleep late, and I asked them not to wake her up. It took a few reminders until everyone knew not to try to get her up for breakfast. The staff would look into her room to check how she was doing and let her sleep.

How does medication management work? Who handles medication renewal? When is a family-filled option used?

Assisted living facilities do not employ medically trained staff. Thus, they are not trained to dispense medications. My mother's assisted living facility worked with a pharmacy that dispensed blister packs for each customer with all their prescription medications combined in a daily pack. Unfortunately, my mother's prescription insurance did not include the pharmacy they were using as their preferred provider. If I wanted medicine to be covered by insurance, I had to be in charge of renewing and picking up prescriptions, then filling the daily medication cassettes myself. This procedure is called the family-filled medication option.

The cassettes were stored in a locked box in my mother's room. The staff would offer the medications to my mother on a schedule prescribed by the doctor. If she did not take medicine in their presence, then they would put the pills back in the locked box and make a notation in the daily report.

Tip:

Ask what pharmacy the assisted living facility is using and then call your insurance and check if your insurance covers the assisted living facility's preferred pharmacy. My mother's insurance did not cover the facility's pharmacy and I had to use family-filled option.

How does the facility handle the situation when the resident refuses to take medication?

The only thing the staff could do about medication refusal was to make a note of it on her record and report to me. Then, it was up to me to convince her that taking medicine was something she had to do for her own benefit.

How long has this facility been in operation?

Is it part of a chain of facilities? If so, where are the other facilities located?

Is there a personal emergency system? (e.g., Lifeline)

In my mother's assisted living, each resident had a pendant. When the resident pressed a button on a pendant, it indicated that one of the staff members needed to come to their room or find them wherever they were. My mother never got used to the pendant; she did not remember what it was for and often lost it. The attendants had a note in my mom's file that she was not aware of how to use it. The only time we used her pendant was when I used it to request that someone open the medical chest for me to refill her medicine cassette. An attendant came to her room within 5 minutes.

Has any resident been asked to leave? What were the reasons?

*Communication with
assisted living facility staff*

Can I communicate with the staff via email?

I found communication via email very helpful. I work in an environment that is not private, and email allowed me to discuss topics that I did not want everyone to hear.

Who do I contact in case of emergency?

I had several emails, cell phones, and phone numbers that I could contact in case of an emergency.

References for the assisted living facility

The most accurate references you can get is by talking to the children of the residents. I stopped a few of them in the parking lot, and, each time, they were eager to share their experiences, both positive and negative.

I also tried to talk to a few residents. Most of the time, the residents were not alone, but with a staff member, so I was not sure if they would tell me anything negative.

Walking around the facility and observing residents was very useful. In some facilities, many residents were just sitting in their wheelchairs in the hallway. In other facilities, they were more alert and doing various things in different parts of the facility. Make a note of what activities are going on and how involved the residents are in the activities.

Make a note of how clean the facility is; how it smells. When I was evaluating the rooms, I looked at vacant rooms and occupied rooms. The empty rooms were useful for taking measurements and looking at the details. The occupied rooms were helpful to see if housekeeping was doing a good job keeping the place clean.

Pay attention to how staff members talk to the residents. Do they know their names? Does it look like they know something specific about them? Do they sound friendly and respectful?

QUESTIONS TO ASK WHEN SELECTING NURSING HOMES

When I was choosing the assisted living facility, I also requested to visit the nursing home associated with the assisted living facility. I did so for several places, so that I had some basis for comparison. The most significant difference between different nursing homes was in how the residents looked and behaved. In some nursing homes, the residents looked sedated. I was particularly struck by one place where all residents were lined up in their wheelchairs in the hallway and were all dozing. In other facilities, the residents were moving around and more engaged.

You need to ask many of the same questions for both assisted living and nursing homes, even if they are associated. In many cases, the answers to the same questions were different.

Questions about the rooms in the nursing home

What is the room and board fee? Are all rooms double occupancy rooms?

In my mother's nursing home, there are only a couple of single rooms. The small number of single rooms is because Medicaid only covers double rooms. The single rooms were reserved for private pay residents.

Is there a separate dementia unit?

My mother's nursing home has a separate dementia unit for advanced dementia patients. It has advanced security to prevent residents from leaving the facility without supervision. In my mother's area, there is some minimal security as well. For example, the elevator requires a special code for the elevator door to open. This security code prevents the residents from accidentally going to another floor and getting lost.

Is a phone line provided, and if there is a phone fee?

My mother's nursing home does not provide a phone. There is a phone jack next to the bed, but it is the resident's responsibility to install and pay for the phone.

Is TV and cable provided and is there a fee?

TV and cable are provided and are part of the basic room and board fee. My mother does not enjoy watching TV, so she asked the TV to be removed. Removing the TV gave her extra space on the dresser. Even though TV was removed her cost of the room did not change.

Questions about selecting the room in the nursing home

Is there a choice of rooms?

I did not have a choice of rooms. I could specify my mother's preference for the window side of the room. There was no guarantee that her preference could be accommodated.

What furniture is provided?

The room included a bed, a dresser, and a wardrobe. I asked if my mother could bring her own bed, and the answer was no. All beds are adjustable hospital-style beds with sidebars that could be lowered.

Tip:

Bring a measuring tape to measure empty wall space. Most of the furniture in the nursing home room was provided, yet there was still some room to bring in some favorite personal furniture such as a chair or a small table. My mother enjoyed sitting at the table for meals and reading. The table she had in the assisted living was too large to fit in the space available in the nursing home room. However, after get-

ting the exact measurements of the free wall space, I was able to find a small table that did fit. Keeping some old habits has been comforting for her.

Does the room have a microwave oven?

No. The rooms have no kitchen area. The rooms have no microwave oven and no refrigerator.

Can a resident eat in their room if they wish?

Yes. If my mother forgets to go to dinner or lunch, the staff brings the food to her.

Will the food be brought to the room on the resident request?

Yes, some residents have all of their meals in their own room.

Questions about the nursing home facility

How many staff members are in the facility during the day, evening, weekend

Is there a hair salon on the premises?

Is there a library?

My mother's nursing home did not have a library; however, my mother was able ask for books from the activity coordinator. The selection is not as good as in the assisted living facility and I brought additional reading material.

What activities are provided for the residents? Are the residents required to take part in activities if they don't wish to participate?

I observed people playing bingo and word games daily. My mother did not take part in games.

Can the kitchen handle special food prep, for example, chopping food for every meal for someone with dentures?

Food prep has not been a problem. My mother said

the food is prepared well, and she has no trouble eating it.

How long has this facility been in operation?

Is there a personal emergency system? (e.g., Lifeline pendants)

There are no lifeline pendants. Each bed is equipped with an emergency button.

Who does the laundry?

In the nursing home, I did the laundry for all personal items. The nursing home does laundry for the bedding.

Is there a doctor, dentist, and podiatrist associated with the facility?

There are several doctors associated with the facility. I received a bill from a dentist that visited my mother, and the bill included a charge for a home visit.

How does medication management work? Who renews prescriptions?

The nursing home takes care of medication management. In fact, they cannot accept any medication provided by the family. The medication left over from her time in the assisted living facility had to be thrown out; the nursing home could not take any of the medicine she already had.

Does this facility accept Medicaid?

The nursing homes I visited all accepted Medicaid. Since it is a critical question for residents who might ran out of money, it is best to be sure that the facility does accept Medicaid.

How often are the residents bathed?

My mother's nursing home offers showers twice a week. The residents can accept the offer to shower or reject it. When my mother rejected the shower offer several times in a row, the social worker contacted me and asked me to talk to my mother about the showers. She also offered me an option to have my mother take her showers while I was visiting, if I thought my mother would be more comfortable doing it when I was there.

Communication with the nursing home staff

Can I communicate with the staff via email?

Communication in the nursing home has not been as good as in the assisted living facility. I could communicate with the social worker using email. She was able to check if my mother disconnected her phone and other minor things like that. I could also use email to talk to the business manager about bills. I could not communicate with the nursing staff via email. I could call them, but a few times I called, I felt they were rushing as we spoke.

Who can I contact in case of an emergency?

The emergency contact is the nurse's desk on my mother's floor.

CONCLUSION

If I knew the things that I know now about the process, it would have been a lot easier and less stressful for me to find the right home for my mother. I hope I've been able to help you by sharing my story and the steps and lessons I have learned along the way. My wish is to make it easier for you to navigate the maze of rules, forms, and deadlines and make confident decisions of what is best for your loved ones. I wish you well!

If you would like to receive questions listed in this book as a spreadsheet, feel free to email me at kadydash@outlook.com, and I will be happy to email it to you.

If you found this book helpful, please leave a review on Amazon. Amazon ranks search results based on review ratings and keywords in the reviews. Your review can help other people in similar situations find and benefit from this book. Thank you!

APPENDIX

This appendix contains links to all of the documents that I needed when helping my mother get Medicaid in the Commonwealth of Massachusetts. Be aware that while all links were current at the time of publication, many forms are updated annually. These links are only provided for your reference. Make sure that you use the latest available version of any forms and for the state where you live.

• Medicaid is a federal program, so various state programs have a lot in common. My experience with the Massachusetts Medicaid system should be helpful and relevant to other programs. For details and application for your specific state, please refer to

https://www.medicaid.gov/state-overviews/index.html

• Regulations that specify requirements for people to be eligible for Medicaid

130 CMR 456.00: Long-term care services

https://www.mass.gov/regulations/130-CMR-45600-long-term-care-services

130 CMR 408.00: Adult foster care

https://www.mass.gov/regulations/130-CMR-40800-adult-foster-care

• The link to the application for Medicaid for Massachusetts is below. In the Commonwealth of Massachusetts, Medicaid is called Mass Health. You can find applications for other states by using the state name and the word Medicaid as keywords.

https://www.benefits.gov/benefit/1282

• If you live in Massachusetts use the form below to request information about your accounts from a financial institution. When you use this form, the financial institution will not charge a research fee:

https://www.mass.gov/files/documents/2016/07/pv/fir-1.pdf

According to Massachusetts General Law c. 118E, §

23A MassHealth (Medicaid) applicant is entitled to this information free of charge. If you live in a different state check if your legislature has a similar law.

• Below is a statute that prohibits requiring a family member to be a guarantor of payments:

Admission, transfer, and discharge rights. The admission policy section of 42 CFR 483.12(d)(2)

https://www.govinfo.gov/content/pkg/CFR-2010-title42-vol5/pdf/CFR-2010-title42-vol5-sec483-12.pdf

• The following three forms must be submitted by the Massachuetts-based nursing home to the Medicaid office when a nursing home resident applies for Medicaid.

Status Change form (SC1):

https://www.mass.gov/files/documents/2016/07/td/status-change-ltc.pdf

Permission to share form (PSI form):

https://www.mass.gov/lists/hipaa-forms-for-masshealth-members

PNA form:

https://www.mass.gov/files/documents/2018/03/22/ltc-112.pdf

• If a person receives Medicaid, they can apply for a discounted phone service called Lifeline.

Lifeline information and prices for all US states on Verizon site:

verizon.com/lifeline

Lifeline federal program information:

https://www.fcc.gov/consumers/guides/lifeline-support-affordable-communications

Lifeline application on Verizon site:

https://www.verizon.com/cs/groups/public/d

• Medicaid laws related to long-term care in a nursing home in the state of Massachusetts:

https://www.nolo.com/legal-encyclopedia/
when-medicaid-massachusetts-will-pay-long-
term-care-nursing-home.html

• Senior Whole Health is one of the Medicare Advantage plans. The first link is to all Medicare Advantage plans, the second link is specific to Senior Whole Health in Massachusetts.

All Medicare Advantage plans:

https://q1medicare.com/PartD-
GoogleWebSearchGoogleWebSearchGo.php?
cx=partner-pub-9185979746634162%3Afhatcw-
ivsf&cof=FORID
%3A10&ie=ISO-8859-1&q=2020+Medicare
+Advantage+Plan+Benefit+&sa=Search

Massachusetts Senior Whole Health plan:

https://q1medicare.com/MedicareAdvantage-
PartC-MedicareHealthPlanBenefits.php?
state=MA&source=2016MAFinder&ZIP=&countyC
ode=25027&contractId=H2224&planId=001&seg
mentId=0&plan=Senior%20Whole%20Health
%20(HMO%20SNP)%20-
%20H2224-001-0&utm_source=partd&utm_medi
um=mafinder&utm_campaign=enrollbutton

• Can a nursing home resident be evicted? This issue is addressed in Transfer and Discharges from a Nursing Home and Your Rights:

https://ctlawhelp.org/en/nursing-home-transfers-discharges

SUMMARY OF DOCUMENTS YOU WILL NEED

Y ou need to have a full understanding of your parent's financial resources and have legal documents to be able to manage these resources on your parent's behalf. Try to obtain this information and these documents while your parent is well.

• Durable Power of attorney

• Health care proxy document that identifies a health-care agent

- Social security id

- Medicare id

- Health insurance information

- Disability and Long term insurance information

- Access to the safety deposit box

- Tax return records for the last three years

- Five-year record for all investments (banks, mutual funds, stocks, bonds, etc.). This record should cover both purchases and sales.

- A living will, a document that identifies your parent's wishes about medical decisions, is not required but would be helpful to any caregiver.

HOW TO FIND CARE FOR YOUR ELDERLY PARENT

- Information about real estate sales

ALPHABETICAL INDEX

A Place for Mom   3, 12
Assisted Living   1, 8, 10pp., 14pp., 18, 20pp., 30, 32, 50,
   65pp., 72p., 75pp., 82, 85pp., 90
Bills   6, 38pp., 51, 56p., 87
Dementia   5p., 8, 11, 16, 18, 23p., 32, 39, 52p., 67, 71, 82
Guarantor   20pp., 25, 31, 69, 89
Health care proxy   9, 92
Medicaid   3, 10p., 16, 25, 29, 31, 34pp., 45pp., 49p., 52pp.,
   59pp., 70, 82, 86p., 89p., 92
Medications   8, 18p., 32, 63, 78
Nursing Home   1, 3p., 8, 11, 14, 16, 18p., 21p., 25pp.,
   29pp., 33pp., 37pp., 45, 48, 56, 60p., 63, 65, 69p., 73, 82pp.,
   90p.
Nursing homes   8, 16, 21, 65, 69, 82
Power of attorney   3, 9, 31, 37, 44, 50pp., 55, 92
Questions   5, 8, 10, 22, 32, 38, 43, 58, 65p., 72p., 81pp., 85

BOOKS BY THIS AUTHOR

Back Surgery: Step By Step Recovery Guide

Are you facing back surgery? This book will supplement the medical information provided by your doctor. Be prepared to have a faster and easier recovery from back surgery.

Learn about:

ITEMS to bring to the hospital and rehabilitation facility
16 mobility tools that will make rehabilitation easier
11 physical therapy exercises that ARE most effective for recovery
A realistic expectation of pain and limitations during recovery

This is what readers are saying:

"I did NOT find anything like this book - a true, honest first-hand account of the trials and tribulations of back surgery from a recovery perspective. I wish I had; there was a lot of good information gathered in one place that I had spent hours and days researching and compiling from various online resources." By John M. Vizcarra

"One would think tackling this subject should inevitably be sad or boring or both - not so!"Back Surgery" story is told with humor - great feature to have when you are subjected to all these small indignities of dependent existence. It has this admirable attitude not of a victim, but of a fighter and a very intelligent no-nonsense fighter." By Irina Khasin

"... rather than a cleaned-up idealized version, she hopes to guide and inform the reader about what to actually expect from surgery. This book should be required reading for anyone contemplating having back surgery." By Joe Veilleux

Show Some Spine: The Most Effective Physical Therapy Exercises For A Strong Back

The author spent many months doing supervised physical therapy exercises for lower back pain. This book is a collection of exercises and instructions

that she found to be most effective in her rehabilitation. In our busy lives sometimes it is hard to find time to exercise. If you only have a few minutes a day to exercise "Show Some Spine" and make these ten exercises part of your day. Your back will thank you!

This is what readers are saying:

"I was is pain(an outbreak of a recurring problem) and in desperation I bought this book. The exercises are realistically pitched - not over ambitious - and I felt an improvement very quickly. " By DOB

"What I like best about this effort is that it is written by an author who has actually learned the techniques as a patient rather than a provider. ... so there isn't any theoretical fluff here, just simple exercises that will help to reduce, and potentially eliminate, back pain over the long haul. The illustrations and explanations are fully adequate to explain the basic motions." By D. Buxman

"As a veteran and an expert in physical fitness who overcame both severe neck and back pains myself, I can tell the exercises introduced in this book are really helpful if employed correctly and consistently with patience." By Young H.D. Kim

www.ingramcontent.com/pod-product-compliance
Lightning Source LLC
Chambersburg PA
CBHW070646220526
45466CB00001B/312